LIVING WITH CONGESTIVE HEART FAILURE

A Comprehensive Guide to Thriving with Congestive Heart Failure

DR. THOMAS FELAN

<u>Disclaimer</u>

The information provided in this book is for educational and informational purposes only. It is not intended as a substitute for professional medical advice, diagnosis, or treatment. Always seek the advice of your physician or other qualified healthcare provider with any questions you may have regarding a medical condition or treatment.

The content of this book is based on general knowledge and research available up to the time of its publication. Health and medical information are subject to constant advancements and changes. Therefore, the author, publisher, and any contributors to this book make no representations or warranties of any kind, express or implied, regarding the accuracy, completeness, suitability, or applicability of the information contained herein.

Readers are encouraged to consult their healthcare providers before making any changes to their diet, exercise routines, or medical treatment plans. Individual responses to dietary and lifestyle changes can vary, and what works for one person may not work for another.

The author and publisher of this book are not responsible for any adverse effects, injuries, or damages arising from the information provided within these pages. Any reliance you place on the information in this book is strictly at your own risk.

Please consult your healthcare provider before beginning any new dietary or exercise program, making changes to your existing treatment plan, or relying on the information presented in this book. Your healthcare provider is the best source of information regarding your individual health situation.

By reading and utilizing the information in this book, you agree to the terms of this disclaimer. If you do not agree with these terms, please refrain from using this book.

Remember that the field of health and medicine is complex and rapidly evolving. The information in this book is not a substitute for professional medical advice, and readers should always prioritize their health and safety by consulting qualified healthcare professionals.

Table of content

Introduction

Welcome to "Living with Congestive Heart Failure," a guide crafted with compassion and expertise to empower you on your journey towards a heart-healthy life. In these pages, we embark on a voyage through understanding the intricacies of congestive heart failure (CHF) and navigating the path to a fulfilling and vibrant existence despite its challenges.

This book is not just a compendium of medical insights; it's a beacon of hope, offering practical strategies, emotional support, and a roadmap for transforming the challenges of CHF into opportunities for a richer life. Whether you're newly diagnosed, supporting a loved one, or seeking to enhance your understanding, this comprehensive guide is designed to be your trusted companion.

As we delve into the complexities of CHF, we invite you to embrace a holistic approach that extends beyond medical interventions. Together, let's explore the profound impact of lifestyle choices, uncover the latest advancements in treatment, and discover the resilience of the human spirit in the face of adversity.

With each turn of the page, may you find not only valuable information but also inspiration to live a heart-healthy life filled with joy, purpose, and a renewed sense of well-being. Welcome to a journey where knowledge becomes empowerment, and

every chapter unfolds a new opportunity for
a brighter tomorrow.

Understanding Congestive Heart Failure

Congestive Heart Failure, often abbreviated as CHF, is a chronic and progressive condition where the heart's ability to pump blood is compromised, leading to an insufficient supply of oxygen and nutrients to the body's tissues. Contrary to a common misconception, CHF does not mean that the heart has stopped working; rather, it is struggling to meet the body's demands efficiently.

Mechanisms of Heart Failure:
- CHF can result from various heart conditions that weaken the heart muscle or make it work too hard. Common causes include coronary

artery disease, myocardial infarction (heart attack), hypertension, and valvular heart diseases. Over time, these factors contribute to the heart's reduced pumping capacity.

Left vs. Right Heart Failure:

- CHF can affect the left side, right side, or both chambers of the heart. Left heart failure typically leads to pulmonary congestion, causing symptoms like shortness of breath, while right heart failure results in systemic congestion, leading to fluid retention and swelling in the extremities.

Symptoms and Warning Signs:

Recognizing the signs of CHF is crucial for early intervention. Common symptoms include fatigue, shortness of breath (especially during physical activity or when lying down), persistent coughing, fluid retention causing swelling in the legs and abdomen, and a rapid or irregular heartbeat.

Diagnostic Tests:

Accurate diagnosis is pivotal for effective management. Healthcare providers may employ various tests, including echocardiograms, electrocardiograms (ECG or EKG), chest X-rays, and blood tests to evaluate heart function, identify underlying causes, and determine the most appropriate treatment plan.

Stages of Heart Failure:

CHF is often categorized into stages based on the severity of symptoms and limitations. Understanding these stages helps guide treatment strategies and lifestyle adjustments, emphasizing the importance of proactive management to prevent progression.

Risk Factors:

Certain factors increase the risk of developing CHF, including age, family history, obesity, diabetes, and lifestyle choices such as smoking and excessive alcohol consumption. Recognizing and addressing these risk factors is crucial for prevention and long-term management.

Comorbidities and Complications:

CHF is often accompanied by other health conditions, such as kidney problems or diabetes. Additionally, if left unmanaged, it can lead to serious complications, including arrhythmias, heart valve issues, and, in severe cases, multi-organ failure.

Understanding Congestive Heart Failure involves not only grasping the physiological aspects of the condition but also appreciating the profound impact it has on an individual's quality of life. In the subsequent sections of this guide, we will delve into the diverse aspects of managing CHF, from lifestyle modifications to advanced medical interventions, with the ultimate goal of empowering you to navigate this journey with knowledge and resilience.

Importance of Managing CHF

Congestive Heart Failure is a chronic condition that demands vigilant management to enhance quality of life, slow disease progression, and reduce the risk of complications. The significance of proactive management extends beyond alleviating symptoms; it involves a holistic approach addressing physical, emotional, and lifestyle aspects.

Enhancing Quality of Life:
Effective management of CHF can significantly improve the overall well-being of individuals. By optimizing heart function and minimizing symptoms like shortness of breath and fatigue, individuals can regain a

sense of normalcy and actively participate in daily activities.

Preventing Disease Progression:

CHF is a progressive condition, meaning it tends to worsen over time. However, with appropriate medical interventions, lifestyle modifications, and adherence to prescribed treatments, it is possible to slow down the progression of the disease, preserving heart function and minimizing complications.

Reducing Hospitalizations:

Unmanaged CHF often leads to recurrent hospitalizations due to exacerbations and complications. By actively managing the condition, individuals can reduce the frequency and severity of these episodes, promoting stability and reducing the economic and emotional burden associated with hospital stays.

Minimizing Complications:

CHF is associated with various complications, including arrhythmias, kidney problems, and increased risk of stroke. Proactive management helps mitigate these complications through measures such as medication management, regular monitoring, and lifestyle adjustments.

Empowering Self-Care:

Managing CHF involves active participation from individuals in their own care. This empowerment includes adhering to medication regimens, adopting heart-healthy lifestyles, monitoring symptoms, and promptly seeking medical attention when needed. This engagement fosters a sense of control and self-efficacy.

Addressing Emotional Well-being:

Living with CHF can be emotionally challenging. Effective management not only focuses on physical aspects but also considers the emotional impact of the condition. Support from healthcare providers, counselors, and support groups can contribute to improved mental health and resilience.

Optimizing Medication Management:

Medications play a crucial role in managing CHF by improving heart function, reducing symptoms, and preventing complications. Adhering to prescribed medication regimens is paramount to achieving optimal outcomes.

Encouraging Lifestyle Modifications:

Heart-healthy lifestyle choices, including a balanced diet, regular exercise, and smoking cessation, are integral to CHF management. These lifestyle modifications not only support heart health but also contribute to overall well-being.

Improving Long-Term Prognosis:

The long-term prognosis for individuals with CHF is influenced by the quality of management. By actively addressing the condition, individuals can enhance their life expectancy and enjoy a higher quality of life.

Importance of managing Congestive Heart Failure lies in the opportunity to lead a fulfilling life despite the challenges posed by the condition. Through a comprehensive and collaborative approach between individuals, healthcare providers, and support networks, effective CHF management can be a transformative journey towards improved health and well-being.

Causes and Risk Factors

Congestive Heart Failure (CHF) arises from a multitude of factors that affect the heart's ability to pump blood effectively. Understanding both the causes and risk factors is crucial for early identification, prevention, and comprehensive management of this chronic condition.

Coronary Artery Disease (CAD):
The most common cause of CHF is coronary artery disease, a condition where the blood vessels supplying the heart muscle become narrowed or blocked. Reduced blood flow to the heart muscle can lead to damage and weaken the heart over time.
Myocardial Infarction (Heart Attack):

A heart attack, resulting from a sudden blockage of blood flow to a part of the heart, can cause damage to the heart muscle. This damage may impair the heart's ability to pump blood effectively, contributing to the development of CHF.

Hypertension (High Blood Pressure):
- Chronic high blood pressure forces the heart to work harder to pump blood against increased resistance. This sustained strain on the heart muscle can lead to its weakening over time, ultimately contributing to heart failure.

Valvular Heart Diseases:
- Malfunctioning heart valves, either due to congenital conditions or acquired diseases, can disrupt normal

blood flow within the heart. Over time, this can result in heart failure, particularly if left untreated.

Cardiomyopathies:

- Conditions that directly affect the heart muscle, such as dilated cardiomyopathy or hypertrophic cardiomyopathy, can lead to CHF. These disorders often result in structural changes that compromise the heart's ability to pump blood effectively.

Diabetes Mellitus:

- Diabetes, especially when poorly controlled, is a significant risk factor for developing CHF. The metabolic changes associated with diabetes can contribute to both coronary artery disease and direct damage to the heart muscle.

Obesity:

- Excess body weight puts strain on the heart, leading to an increased risk of heart failure. Obesity is often associated with other risk factors such as hypertension and diabetes, further compounding its impact on heart health.

Smoking:

- Tobacco smoke contains chemicals that can damage blood vessels and heart tissue. Smoking is a modifiable risk factor, and quitting can significantly reduce the risk of developing CHF and other cardiovascular diseases.

Genetic Predisposition:

- Family history plays a role in heart health. Individuals with a family history of heart failure may have a genetic predisposition to the condition, highlighting the importance of regular screenings and lifestyle modifications.

Alcohol and Substance Abuse:

- Excessive alcohol consumption and substance abuse can contribute to heart muscle damage and increase the risk of developing heart failure. Moderation and abstinence are essential in managing these risk factors.

Understanding the causes and risk factors of Congestive Heart Failure provides a foundation for preventive measures and early intervention. By addressing modifiable risk factors through lifestyle changes, medication adherence, and regular medical check-ups, individuals can reduce their susceptibility to CHF and work towards maintaining a heart-healthy lifestyle.

Heart Conditions Leading to CHF

Various heart conditions can pave the way to Congestive Heart Failure (CHF), a complex and chronic condition characterized by the heart's diminished ability to pump blood effectively. Recognizing these underlying heart conditions is crucial for early intervention and targeted management. Here are some key heart conditions associated with the development of CHF:

Coronary Artery Disease (CAD):

- CAD is a primary contributor to CHF. It involves the narrowing or blockage of coronary arteries, leading to reduced blood flow to the heart muscle. Chronic ischemia (lack of blood supply) can result in myocardial damage and weaken the heart over time, eventually culminating in heart failure.

Myocardial Infarction (Heart Attack):

- A heart attack occurs when blood flow to a part of the heart muscle is abruptly blocked, leading to tissue death. The damage from a heart attack can impair the heart's ability to pump blood efficiently, setting the stage for the development of CHF.

Hypertensive Heart Disease:

- Chronic high blood pressure forces the heart to work harder to pump blood against elevated resistance. Over time, this increased workload can lead to hypertrophy (thickening) of the heart muscle and, subsequently, heart failure.

Valvular Heart Diseases:

- Malfunctioning heart valves, whether due to congenital defects or acquired conditions like rheumatic fever, can disrupt normal blood flow within the heart. This can result in volume overload, eventually causing the heart to weaken and leading to CHF.

Cardiomyopathies:

- Cardiomyopathies are conditions that directly affect the structure and function of the heart muscle. Dilated cardiomyopathy, where the heart chambers become enlarged and weakened, and hypertrophic cardiomyopathy, characterized by abnormal thickening of the heart muscle, are examples that can progress to heart failure.

Arrhythmias:

- Irregular heart rhythms, such as atrial fibrillation or ventricular tachycardia, can contribute to heart failure. Arrhythmias disrupt the heart's coordinated pumping action, leading to inefficient blood circulation and potential weakening of the heart muscle.

Congenital Heart Defects:

- Structural abnormalities present at birth, affecting the heart's chambers, valves, or blood vessels, can contribute to heart failure later in life. These defects may create an additional strain on the heart, leading to progressive deterioration.

Infections of the Heart:

- Infections such as myocarditis or endocarditis can cause inflammation of the heart muscle or inner lining of the heart. Chronic inflammation may lead to structural damage, impairing the heart's ability to function optimally.

Pericardial Diseases:

- Disorders affecting the pericardium, the sac surrounding the heart, can impact the heart's normal function. Conditions like constrictive pericarditis can restrict the heart's ability to pump effectively, contributing to heart failure.

Recognizing and addressing these heart conditions through early detection, medical intervention, and lifestyle modifications are pivotal in preventing or managing CHF. A comprehensive approach that addresses both the underlying heart condition and its impact on heart function is essential for improving outcomes and enhancing the quality of life for individuals at risk of or living with CHF.

Lifestyle Factors

Beyond medical interventions, lifestyle factors play a critical role in managing Congestive Heart Failure (CHF). Adopting heart-healthy habits can enhance overall well-being, alleviate symptoms, and contribute to the prevention of complications. Here are key lifestyle factors to consider:

Dietary Guidelines:

- Heart-Healthy Eating: Emphasize a diet rich in fruits, vegetables, whole grains, lean proteins, and low-fat dairy. Limit saturated and trans fats, cholesterol, and sodium to promote heart health.

- Fluid Intake Management: Monitoring fluid intake is crucial, especially for individuals with CHF experiencing fluid retention. Consistency in fluid consumption is essential to prevent sudden changes in volume.

Exercise and Physical Activity:

- Tailored Exercise Programs: Engage in regular, moderate exercise as recommended by healthcare providers. Customized exercise plans can improve cardiovascular fitness without overexertion.

- Monitoring Activity Levels: Be mindful of physical activity and recognize individual limits. Tracking symptoms like fatigue or shortness of breath during exercise helps maintain a safe and effective fitness routine.

Smoking Cessation:

- Tobacco-Free Lifestyle: Quitting smoking is crucial for heart health. Smoking damages blood vessels and contributes to the progression of heart disease. Support programs and medications can aid in the cessation process.

Alcohol Moderation:

- Limiting Alcohol Intake: Moderation in alcohol consumption is advised, as excessive drinking can contribute to heart muscle damage. Individuals with CHF should consult healthcare providers for personalized recommendations.

Weight Management:

- Maintaining a Healthy Weight: Achieving and maintaining a healthy weight reduces the strain on the heart. Weight management is often a combination of a balanced diet and regular physical activity.

Stress Management:

- Mindfulness and Relaxation Techniques: Chronic stress can negatively impact heart health. Practicing mindfulness, deep breathing, or engaging in activities that promote relaxation can contribute to stress management.

Regular Medical Check-ups:

- Adherence to Medication Regimens: Consistent use of prescribed medications is vital for managing CHF. Regular check-ups with healthcare providers ensure appropriate medication adjustments and monitoring of overall health.

Sleep Hygiene:

- Quality Sleep: Aim for sufficient and restful sleep. Elevated pillows can help reduce nighttime symptoms like shortness of breath. Consult healthcare providers if sleep disturbances persist.

Self-Monitoring:

- Awareness of Symptoms: Regular self-monitoring of symptoms, such as weight changes, swelling, or changes in exercise tolerance, enables early detection of potential issues. Prompt reporting of changes to healthcare providers is crucial.

Social Support:

- Engaging Support Networks: Emotional well-being is integral to heart health. Building a strong support network, including family, friends, and support groups, can provide encouragement and assistance in managing the challenges of CHF.

By integrating these lifestyle factors into daily routines, individuals with CHF can actively contribute to their well-being and improve their overall quality of life. Collaborating with healthcare providers for personalized guidance ensures that lifestyle modifications align with individual health needs and promote effective CHF management.

Genetic Predisposition

Genetic factors can significantly influence an individual's susceptibility to various health conditions, including Congestive Heart Failure (CHF). Understanding genetic predisposition is crucial for identifying risk factors, implementing preventive measures, and tailoring management strategies. Here's an exploration of the connection between genetics and CHF:

Family History:

- Inherited Risk: A family history of heart disease, particularly CHF, can indicate a genetic predisposition. If close relatives, such as parents or siblings, have experienced CHF, it may elevate an individual's risk.

Genetic Variants and Mutations:

- Inherited Mutations: Specific genetic variations or mutations can increase the likelihood of developing heart conditions that may lead to CHF. For example, mutations affecting proteins involved in heart muscle function can impact cardiac health.

Heredity in Cardiac Conditions:

- Congenital Heart Defects: Some genetic factors contribute to congenital heart defects, which, if present at birth, may lead to heart failure later in life. Understanding the genetic basis of these defects informs both prevention and management strategies.

Risk Stratification:

- Genetic Testing: Advances in genetic testing enable individuals to assess their risk of developing certain cardiovascular conditions, including those predisposing to CHF. Genetic testing can identify specific mutations and guide proactive measures.

Polygenic Risk:

- Multiple Genetic Factors: CHF often results from a combination of genetic factors rather than a single gene mutation. Polygenic risk, where multiple genetic variations collectively influence risk, underscores the complexity of genetic predisposition.

Interaction with Environmental Factors:

- Gene-Environment Interplay: Genetic predisposition interacts with environmental factors such as lifestyle, diet, and exposure to toxins. Understanding this interplay helps in crafting comprehensive strategies for CHF prevention and management.

Early Intervention:

- Preventive Measures: Knowledge of genetic predisposition allows for early intervention. Individuals with a family history or identified genetic risk factors can proactively adopt heart-healthy lifestyles, undergo regular screenings, and work closely with healthcare providers for personalized care.

Tailored Treatment Approaches:

- Precision Medicine: Genetic insights contribute to the emerging field of precision medicine. Tailoring treatment plans based on an individual's genetic profile holds promise for optimizing therapeutic interventions and improving outcomes in CHF management.

Genetic Counseling:

- Guidance and Support: Genetic counseling provides individuals and families with information about their genetic risk, implications, and available preventive measures. It offers emotional support and aids in informed decision-making regarding genetic testing and management strategies.

Public Health Implications:

- Population Health Strategies: Understanding genetic predisposition at the population level informs public health initiatives. Identifying high-risk groups allows for targeted interventions, screening programs, and education to reduce the overall burden of CHF.

Genetic predisposition plays a significant role in shaping an individual's risk of developing Congestive Heart Failure. While genetics contribute to susceptibility, lifestyle modifications, early intervention, and collaboration with healthcare providers remain pivotal in mitigating risk, managing the condition effectively, and improving overall heart health.

Diagnosing CHF

Diagnosing Congestive Heart Failure is a comprehensive process that involves a combination of medical history assessment, physical examinations, and various diagnostic tests. Early and accurate diagnosis is critical for initiating timely interventions and improving the management of this chronic condition. Here's an overview of the diagnostic approach for CHF:

Medical History and Physical Examination:
- Symptom Assessment: Healthcare providers begin by evaluating symptoms such as shortness of breath, fatigue, persistent coughing, and swelling in the extremities.

- Medical History: Gathering information about the patient's medical history, including any pre-existing heart conditions, family history of heart disease, and risk factors for CHF.

Blood Tests:

- Biomarker Analysis: Blood tests often include measuring biomarkers like B-type natriuretic peptide (BNP) or N-terminal pro B-type natriuretic peptide (NT-proBNP). Elevated levels can indicate heart failure and help in the diagnostic process.

Imaging Studies:

- Echocardiogram: This ultrasound imaging technique provides real-time images of the heart's structure and function, including the pumping capacity (ejection fraction) and any abnormalities in the heart valves or chambers.

- Chest X-ray: X-ray images can reveal changes in the size and shape of the heart and identify signs of congestion in the lungs, common in CHF patients.

Electrocardiogram (ECG or EKG):

- Heart Rhythm Assessment: ECG records the electrical activity of the heart, helping to identify irregular heart rhythms (arrhythmias) and signs of stress on the heart muscle.

Stress Tests:

- Exercise Stress Test: Monitoring the heart's response to physical exertion helps evaluate its capacity and identify any exercise-induced abnormalities.

Cardiac MRI or CT Scan:

- Detailed Imaging: These advanced imaging techniques provide detailed pictures of the heart's structure and can reveal abnormalities not easily detected by other imaging methods.

Nuclear Heart Scan:

- Myocardial Perfusion Imaging: This test involves injecting a small amount of radioactive material to assess blood flow to the heart muscle, helping identify areas with reduced blood supply.

Holter Monitor or Event Recorder:

- Continuous Monitoring: For individuals with intermittent symptoms, these devices record heart activity over an extended period, aiding in the detection of irregularities not captured during a brief office visit.

Pulmonary Function Tests:

- Assessing Lung Function: These tests may be conducted to evaluate lung function and assess the impact of heart failure on respiratory health.

Coronary Angiography:

- Visualizing Coronary Arteries: In cases where coronary artery disease is suspected, a coronary angiogram may be performed to visualize blood flow in the coronary arteries and identify blockages.

The combination of these diagnostic tools allows healthcare providers to assess the severity of CHF, identify underlying causes, and tailor a management plan to the individual's specific needs. Regular follow-up evaluations and adjustments to the treatment plan are essential for ongoing CHF care. Early diagnosis and a multidisciplinary approach involving cardiology, internal medicine, and other healthcare professionals contribute to effective CHF management and improved patient outcomes.

Symptoms and Warning Signs

Recognizing the symptoms and warning signs of Congestive Heart Failure (CHF) is crucial for early intervention and effective management. These indicators may vary among individuals, but common signs include:

Shortness of Breath (Dyspnea):

- Difficulty breathing, especially during physical activity or when lying down.
- Sudden onset of breathlessness may indicate acute exacerbation.

Fatigue and Weakness:

- Persistent tiredness and a sense of weakness, even with minimal exertion.

Persistent Coughing:

- Chronic or worsening cough, often accompanied by white or pink blood-tinged phlegm. This can be a sign of fluid accumulation in the lungs.

Swelling (Edema):

- Accumulation of fluid leading to swelling, especially in the legs, ankles, or abdomen.
- Sudden weight gain may be indicative of fluid retention.

Rapid or Irregular Heartbeat:

- Palpitations, a fluttering sensation, or a feeling of rapid or irregular heartbeats.

Reduced Exercise Tolerance:

- Inability to tolerate physical activity or a decreased capacity for exercise compared to normal.

Increased Need to Urinate at Night (Nocturia):

- Frequent nighttime urination, potentially due to the redistribution of fluid when lying down.

Sudden Weight Gain:

- Unexplained weight gain, often related to fluid retention, may be a sign of worsening heart failure.

Loss of Appetite and Nausea:

- A decrease in appetite or feelings of nausea, which can result from reduced blood flow to the digestive system.

Difficulty Concentrating or Confusion:

- Impaired cognitive function or confusion, which may be related to decreased blood flow to the brain.

It's essential to note that these symptoms can be indicative of various medical conditions, and their presence does not necessarily confirm CHF. However, if individuals experience a combination of these symptoms, particularly if they worsen over time or are accompanied by risk factors such as hypertension, diabetes, or a family history of heart disease, prompt medical evaluation is advised.

Early diagnosis and intervention significantly improve the outcomes for individuals with CHF. If any of these symptoms are observed, seeking medical attention promptly can lead to timely diagnosis, appropriate treatment, and the development of a comprehensive management plan tailored to the individual's needs. Regular follow-ups with healthcare providers are crucial for ongoing monitoring and adjustment of the treatment plan as needed.

Diagnostic Tests

Diagnosing Congestive Heart Failure (CHF) involves a series of diagnostic tests that provide insights into the heart's structure, function, and overall cardiovascular health. These tests help healthcare providers confirm the presence of CHF, identify its underlying causes, and tailor an appropriate management plan. Here are some key diagnostic tests for CHF:

Blood Tests:

- Biomarker Analysis: Blood tests often include measuring biomarkers such as B-type natriuretic peptide (BNP) or N-terminal pro B-type natriuretic peptide (NT-proBNP). Elevated levels of these markers can indicate heart failure.

Imaging Studies:

- Echocardiogram: This ultrasound test provides real-time images of the heart's chambers, valves, and pumping function. It helps assess the ejection fraction (the percentage of blood pumped out with each heartbeat) and identify structural abnormalities.

- Chest X-ray: X-ray images help evaluate the size and shape of the heart, as well as detect signs of fluid accumulation in the lungs, a common feature in CHF patients.

Electrocardiogram (ECG or EKG):

- Heart Rhythm Assessment: ECG records the electrical activity of the heart, helping identify irregular heart rhythms (arrhythmias) and signs of stress on the heart muscle.

Stress Tests:

- Exercise Stress Test: This test evaluates how the heart responds to physical exertion. It can help identify exercise-induced abnormalities and assess cardiovascular fitness.

Cardiac MRI or CT Scan:

- Detailed Imaging: These advanced imaging techniques provide detailed pictures of the heart's structure and can reveal abnormalities not easily detected by other imaging methods.

Nuclear Heart Scan:

- Myocardial Perfusion Imaging: This test involves injecting a small amount of radioactive material to assess blood flow to the heart muscle. It helps identify areas with reduced blood supply.

Holter Monitor or Event Recorder:

- Continuous Monitoring: For individuals with intermittent symptoms, these devices record heart activity over an extended period, aiding in the detection of irregularities not captured during a brief office visit.

Pulmonary Function Tests:

- Assessing Lung Function: These tests may be conducted to evaluate lung function and assess the impact of heart failure on respiratory health.

Coronary Angiography:

- Visualizing Coronary Arteries: In cases where coronary artery disease is suspected, a coronary angiogram may be performed to visualize blood flow in the coronary arteries and identify blockages.

Tilt Table Test:

- Assessing Blood Pressure Regulation: This test helps evaluate how the heart and nervous system respond to changes in body position, providing insights into potential causes of fainting or dizziness.

B-type Natriuretic Peptide (BNP) Test:

- Specific Biomarker Test: In addition to blood tests, a BNP test may be conducted to measure the levels of this hormone, which increase in response to heart failure.

These diagnostic tests collectively aid in determining the severity of CHF, identifying the underlying causes, and guiding the development of an individualized treatment plan. Regular follow-up assessments and adjustments to the management plan are essential for ongoing care and optimal outcomes for individuals living with CHF.

Treatment Options

The management of Congestive Heart Failure (CHF) involves a comprehensive approach aimed at alleviating symptoms, improving heart function, and enhancing the overall quality of life. Treatment strategies are tailored to individual needs, and they may include the following components:

Medications:

- Diuretics: These medications help reduce fluid buildup by increasing urine output, alleviating symptoms of congestion and swelling.
- ACE Inhibitors (Angiotensin-Converting Enzyme Inhibitors) and ARBs (Angiotensin II

Receptor Blockers): These drugs relax blood vessels, reducing strain on the heart and improving blood flow.

- Beta-Blockers: These medications slow the heart rate and decrease the force of contraction, relieving stress on the heart.

- Aldosterone Antagonists: These drugs help control sodium and fluid balance, preventing fluid retention.

- Digitalis (Digoxin): This medication improves the heart's pumping ability, particularly in cases with reduced ejection fraction.

Lifestyle Modifications:

- Dietary Changes: Adopting a heart-healthy diet low in sodium and saturated fats helps manage fluid retention and supports overall cardiovascular health.

- Regular Exercise: A tailored exercise program improves cardiovascular fitness and helps individuals with CHF better tolerate physical activity.

- Smoking Cessation: Quitting smoking is crucial to improve overall cardiovascular health.

- Limiting Alcohol Intake: Moderation in alcohol consumption is advised to prevent exacerbation of heart failure symptoms.

Device Therapy:

- Implantable Cardioverter-Defibrillator (ICD): For individuals at risk of life-threatening arrhythmias, an ICD may be implanted to monitor and regulate heart rhythm.

- Cardiac Resynchronization Therapy (CRT): This therapy involves the use of a pacemaker to synchronize the contractions of the heart's chambers, improving pumping efficiency.

Surgical Interventions:

- Coronary Artery Bypass Grafting (CABG): In cases of significant coronary artery disease, bypass surgery may be recommended to improve blood flow to the heart muscle.

- Heart Valve Repair or Replacement: Surgical procedures may be performed to repair or replace malfunctioning heart valves.

- Ventricular Assist Devices (VADs): In advanced cases, VADs can be implanted to assist the heart's pumping function while awaiting heart transplantation.

Heart Transplant:

- Transplantation: In severe cases where other treatments are insufficient, heart transplantation may be considered as a last resort.

Education and Support:

- Patient Education: Understanding CHF, its symptoms, and the importance of adhering to prescribed medications and lifestyle changes is crucial for effective self-management.

- Support Groups: Joining support groups provides emotional support, shared experiences, and valuable insights into coping with CHF.

Regular Monitoring and Follow-up:

- Ongoing Assessment: Regular check-ups with healthcare providers involve monitoring symptoms, adjusting medications, and assessing the effectiveness of the treatment plan.
- Self-Monitoring: Individuals are encouraged to monitor their weight, blood pressure, and symptoms at home to detect changes and report them promptly.

The combination of these treatment options allows for a comprehensive and personalized approach to managing CHF. Successful management often involves collaboration between healthcare providers, patients, and, when applicable, caregivers.

Regular communication, adherence to treatment plans, and a proactive approach to lifestyle modifications contribute to improved outcomes and a better quality of life for individuals living with CHF.

Medications

The pharmacological management of Congestive Heart Failure (CHF) aims to alleviate symptoms, improve heart function, and reduce the progression of the condition. Medications prescribed for CHF target various aspects of the cardiovascular system. Here are key classes of medications commonly used in CHF treatment:

Diuretics:

- Function: Diuretics, such as furosemide and hydrochlorothiazide, help the kidneys remove excess fluid from the body, reducing symptoms of congestion and swelling.

- Indication: Used to manage fluid retention and alleviate symptoms like shortness of breath and edema.

ACE Inhibitors (Angiotensin-Converting Enzyme Inhibitors):

- Examples: Enalapril, lisinopril, ramipril.
- Function: ACE inhibitors relax blood vessels, reducing strain on the heart and improving blood flow.
- Indication: Prescribed to manage blood pressure, improve heart function, and prevent further progression of heart failure.

ARBs (Angiotensin II Receptor Blockers):

- Examples: Losartan, valsartan, candesartan.
- Function: Similar to ACE inhibitors, ARBs relax blood vessels, reducing

strain on the heart and improving blood flow.

- Indication: Used in cases where ACE inhibitors may not be tolerated or are contraindicated.

Beta-Blockers:

- Examples: Carvedilol, metoprolol, bisoprolol.

- Function: Beta-blockers slow the heart rate and decrease the force of contraction, reducing the workload on the heart.

- Indication: Prescribed to improve heart function, manage symptoms, and enhance overall cardiovascular health.

Aldosterone Antagonists:

- Examples: Spironolactone, eplerenone.

- Function: These drugs help control sodium and fluid balance, preventing fluid retention and reducing strain on the heart.
- Indication: Used in combination with other medications to manage symptoms and improve outcomes in advanced heart failure.

Digitalis (Digoxin):

- Function: Digoxin improves the heart's pumping ability, particularly in cases with reduced ejection fraction.
- Indication: Prescribed to manage symptoms, especially in cases where other medications may not be sufficient.

Hydralazine and Isosorbide Dinitrate:

- Function: This combination relaxes blood vessels and reduces the heart's workload.
- Indication: Used in specific cases, particularly in individuals with African ancestry or those unable to tolerate ACE inhibitors or ARBs.

Sacubitril/Valsartan (ARNI - Angiotensin Receptor Neprilysin Inhibitor):

- Function: Combines an ARB with a neprilysin inhibitor, enhancing the body's ability to excrete sodium and reducing strain on the heart.
- Indication: Used as an alternative to ACE inhibitors or ARBs in certain cases.

Anticoagulants and Antiplatelet Agents:

- Examples: Warfarin, aspirin, clopidogrel.

- Function: Anticoagulants (blood thinners) and antiplatelet agents reduce the risk of blood clots, which can be a concern in individuals with heart failure.

Statins:

- Examples: Atorvastatin, simvastatin.
- Function: Statins help lower cholesterol levels, managing cardiovascular risk factors.

It's crucial for individuals with CHF to take medications as prescribed, attend regular follow-ups, and communicate with healthcare providers about any changes in symptoms or side effects. Adjustments to medication regimens may be made based on the individual's response and evolving health status. The goal of pharmacological management in CHF is to optimize symptom control, improve quality of life, and slow the progression of the condition.

Lifestyle Changes

Adopting heart-healthy lifestyle changes is integral to the effective management of Congestive Heart Failure (CHF). These modifications aim to improve overall cardiovascular health, alleviate symptoms, and enhance the quality of life for individuals living with CHF. Here are key lifestyle changes recommended for CHF management:

Dietary Modifications:

- Heart-Healthy Eating: Emphasize a diet rich in fruits, vegetables, whole grains, lean proteins, and low-fat dairy. Limit saturated and trans fats, cholesterol, and sodium to support heart health.

- Portion Control: Monitoring portion sizes helps maintain a healthy weight and prevent overeating.

Fluid Intake Management:

- Daily Monitoring: Individuals with CHF, especially those prone to fluid retention, should monitor and regulate their fluid intake. Consistency in fluid consumption helps prevent sudden changes in volume.

Salt Restriction:

- Low-Sodium Diet: Reduce salt intake to manage fluid retention and lower blood pressure. Avoiding processed and packaged foods, which often contain high sodium levels, is crucial.

Regular Exercise:

- Tailored Exercise Program: Engage in regular, moderate exercise as recommended by healthcare providers. Customized exercise plans improve cardiovascular fitness without overexertion.

- Consistent Activity: Consistency in physical activity is vital. Individuals should listen to their bodies and adjust exercise intensity based on their tolerance.

Smoking Cessation:

- Tobacco-Free Lifestyle: Quitting smoking is crucial for heart health. Smoking damages blood vessels and contributes to the progression of heart disease.
- Smoking Cessation Programs: Support programs and medications can aid individuals in their journey to quit smoking.

Limiting Alcohol Intake:

- Moderation: If consuming alcohol, do so in moderation. Excessive alcohol can contribute to heart muscle damage and worsen heart failure symptoms.

Weight Management:

- Maintaining a Healthy Weight: Achieving and maintaining a healthy weight reduces the strain on the heart. Weight management is often a combination of a balanced diet and regular physical activity.

Stress Management:

- Relaxation Techniques: Chronic stress negatively impacts heart health. Practices such as mindfulness, deep breathing, and engaging in activities that promote relaxation are beneficial.

- Prioritizing Mental Health: Emotional well-being is crucial. Seeking support from mental health professionals or support groups can help manage stress and anxiety.

Regular Medical Check-ups:

- Medication Adherence: Consistent use of prescribed medications is vital for managing CHF. Regular check-ups with healthcare providers ensure appropriate medication adjustments and overall health monitoring.

Sleep Hygiene:

- Quality Sleep: Aim for sufficient and restful sleep. Elevated pillows can help reduce nighttime symptoms like shortness of breath. Consult healthcare providers if sleep disturbances persist.

Self-Monitoring:

- Awareness of Symptoms: Regular self-monitoring of symptoms, such as weight changes, swelling, or changes in exercise tolerance, enables early detection of potential issues. Prompt reporting of changes to healthcare providers is crucial.

Social Support:

- Engaging Support Networks: Building a strong support network, including family, friends, and support groups, provides emotional encouragement and assistance in managing the challenges of CHF.

Adopting these lifestyle changes requires commitment and ongoing effort. Working closely with healthcare providers and, when applicable, involving family members or caregivers in the process enhances the effectiveness of these modifications. Tailoring lifestyle changes to individual preferences and health needs contributes to a holistic approach in managing CHF and promotes a better quality of life.

Surgical Interventions

In certain cases of Congestive Heart Failure (CHF), surgical interventions may be recommended to address underlying structural issues, improve blood flow, or provide mechanical support to the heart. Surgical procedures play a crucial role in managing advanced CHF and enhancing the overall quality of life. Here are key surgical interventions commonly employed in CHF management:

Coronary Artery Bypass Grafting (CABG):
- Purpose: CABG is performed to restore blood flow to the heart muscle in cases where coronary arteries are significantly narrowed or blocked. It

involves bypassing blocked arteries using grafts from other blood vessels.

- Indication: Recommended for individuals with CHF caused by coronary artery disease (CAD).

Heart Valve Repair or Replacement:

- Purpose: Repair or replacement of malfunctioning heart valves improves blood flow and reduces the workload on the heart. Valve repair preserves the natural valve, while replacement involves using mechanical or biological prosthetics.
- Indication: Addressing valvular heart diseases contributing to CHF.

Ventricular Assist Devices (VADs):

- Purpose: VADs are mechanical devices implanted to assist the heart's pumping function. They can be used as a bridge to heart transplantation or as destination therapy for individuals ineligible for transplantation.

- Indication: Recommended for advanced CHF with significantly reduced heart function.

Cardiac Resynchronization Therapy (CRT):

- Purpose: CRT involves implanting a pacemaker with specialized leads to synchronize the contractions of the heart's chambers (ventricles). This improves the heart's pumping efficiency.

- Indication: Used to treat heart failure with reduced ejection fraction and electrical dyssynchrony.

Implantable Cardioverter-Defibrillator (ICD):

- Purpose: ICDs monitor heart rhythms and deliver electrical shocks to restore normal rhythm in case of life-threatening arrhythmias.
- Indication: Recommended for individuals at high risk of sudden cardiac death due to arrhythmias.

Heart Transplantation:

- Purpose: Heart transplantation involves replacing a diseased heart with a healthy donor heart.
- Indication: Considered for individuals with end-stage heart failure refractory to other treatments. Eligibility is based on various factors, including overall health and suitability for transplantation.

Ablation Therapy:

- Purpose: Ablation involves using heat or cold energy to destroy or isolate abnormal heart tissue causing arrhythmias.
- Indication: Used to treat specific arrhythmias contributing to heart failure symptoms.

Left Ventricular Assist Device (LVAD):

- Purpose: Similar to VADs, LVADs specifically support the left ventricle's pumping function.
- Indication: Used as a bridge to transplant or as destination therapy in advanced heart failure.

These surgical interventions are often reserved for individuals with advanced CHF who have not responded to other treatments. The decision to undergo surgery is made based on a thorough assessment of the individual's overall health, specific heart condition, and the potential benefits of the procedure.

Surgical interventions can significantly improve symptoms, enhance functional capacity, and extend life for individuals with advanced CHF. Careful evaluation and collaboration between the patient and a multidisciplinary healthcare team guide the selection of the most appropriate surgical approach.

Managing Daily Life with CHF

Living with Congestive Heart Failure (CHF) requires a comprehensive approach to daily life that encompasses medical management, lifestyle modifications, and emotional well-being. Successfully navigating daily life with CHF involves adapting to a new normal and actively participating in self-care. Here are key aspects to consider for effective CHF management:

Medication Adherence:

- Consistent Medication Schedule: Adhering to prescribed medications is crucial. Establish a routine for taking medications as directed by healthcare providers.

- Communication with Healthcare Team: Report any side effects or concerns promptly to healthcare providers. Regular check-ups help assess medication effectiveness and may lead to adjustments.

Dietary Management:

- Low-Sodium Diet: Maintain a low-sodium diet to manage fluid retention. Avoid processed foods and restaurant meals, as they often contain high levels of sodium.
- Portion Control: Practice portion control to prevent overeating and maintain a healthy weight.

Fluid Intake Monitoring:

- Daily Fluid Limits: Individuals with CHF may need to monitor and limit their daily fluid intake. Consistency in fluid consumption is vital to prevent sudden changes in volume.

Regular Exercise:

- Tailored Exercise Program: Engage in regular, moderate exercise as recommended by healthcare providers. Follow a customized exercise plan that suits individual fitness levels and health status.

- Listen to Your Body: Pay attention to how your body responds to exercise, and adjust intensity or duration accordingly. Rest as needed to prevent overexertion.

Symptom Monitoring:

- Daily Self-Assessment: Regularly monitor symptoms such as shortness of breath, fatigue, and swelling.

Report any changes promptly to healthcare providers.

- Use of Self-Monitoring Tools: Keep track of weight, blood pressure, and symptoms using tools recommended by healthcare providers.

Sleep Hygiene:

- Elevated Pillows: For those experiencing nighttime symptoms like shortness of breath, using elevated pillows can help improve sleep quality.
- Addressing Sleep Disturbances: Consult healthcare providers if sleep disturbances persist.

Stress Management:

- Relaxation Techniques: Practice stress-reducing activities such as deep breathing, meditation, or engaging in hobbies.

- Prioritize Mental Health: Addressing emotional well-being is integral to overall health. Seek support from friends, family, or mental health professionals.

Social Support:

- Engaging Support Networks: Build a strong support network that includes family, friends, and support groups. Emotional support is essential for navigating the challenges of CHF.

- Communicate with Loved Ones: Keep loved ones informed about your condition, treatment plan, and any changes in symptoms. Encourage open communication.

Medical Follow-ups:

- Regular Check-ups: Attend regular follow-up appointments with healthcare providers. These visits allow for ongoing assessment, adjustments to the treatment plan, and monitoring of overall health.

- Collaboration with Healthcare Team: Actively participate in discussions with the healthcare team. Share insights about symptoms, lifestyle changes, and any challenges faced.

Emergency Preparedness:

- Know Emergency Signs: Be aware of signs indicating a potential emergency, such as severe shortness of breath or chest pain. Know when to seek immediate medical attention.

- Emergency Contact Information: Keep emergency contact information easily accessible for quick reference.

Adaptation to Physical Limitations:

- Energy Conservation: Prioritize tasks and conserve energy by planning activities during times of peak energy levels.

- Assistive Devices: Use assistive devices, if needed, to facilitate daily activities and reduce strain on the heart.

By actively managing daily life with CHF, individuals can optimize their well-being, minimize symptoms, and enhance their overall quality of life. Consistent communication with healthcare providers, a commitment to self-care, and a supportive network contribute to a successful and fulfilling life while living with CHF.

Dietary Guidelines

A heart-healthy diet is fundamental for managing Congestive Heart Failure (CHF). Dietary choices play a crucial role in controlling symptoms, reducing fluid retention, and supporting overall cardiovascular health. Here are dietary guidelines tailored for individuals living with CHF:

Limit Sodium Intake:

- Daily Sodium Limits: Restrict sodium intake to the level recommended by healthcare providers, typically ranging from 1,500 to 2,300 milligrams per day.
- Avoid Processed Foods: Processed and packaged foods often contain high

levels of sodium. Opt for fresh, whole foods and cook meals at home whenever possible.

Emphasize Heart-Healthy Foods:

- Fruits and Vegetables: Aim for a variety of colorful fruits and vegetables, as they are rich in vitamins, minerals, and antioxidants.
- Whole Grains: Choose whole grains such as brown rice, quinoa, oats, and whole wheat to increase fiber intake.

Portion Control:

- Balanced Meals: Opt for balanced meals that include appropriate portions of lean proteins, whole grains, and vegetables.
- Avoid Overeating: Practice mindful eating and be aware of portion sizes to prevent overeating.

Lean Protein Sources:

- Skinless Poultry, Fish, and Legumes: Choose lean protein sources to support muscle health without adding excessive saturated fats.

- Limit Red Meat: If consuming red meat, choose lean cuts and limit intake.

Healthy Fats:

- Monounsaturated and Polyunsaturated Fats: Include sources like olive oil, avocados, nuts, and seeds, which can contribute to heart health.

- Limit Saturated and Trans Fats: Minimize intake of saturated fats found in fatty meats and full-fat dairy, and avoid trans fats present in processed and fried foods.

Fluid Management:

- Fluid Restrictions: Follow any fluid restrictions prescribed by healthcare providers. Monitor and regulate fluid intake to manage symptoms of fluid retention.
- Limit Caffeine and Alcohol: Both can contribute to dehydration, so moderation is key.

Regular Meal Schedule:

- Consistent Eating Times: Establish a regular eating schedule to help regulate blood sugar levels and prevent overeating.

Monitoring Weight:

- Daily Weight Monitoring: Weighing oneself daily at the same time, using the same scale and under similar conditions, can help detect changes related to fluid retention.

- Prompt Reporting of Changes: Report sudden weight gain to healthcare providers promptly.

Individualized Nutritional Plan:

- Collaboration with a Dietitian: Work with a registered dietitian to create an individualized nutritional plan tailored to specific health needs and dietary restrictions.
- Adjustments as Needed: Periodically reassess and adjust the nutritional plan based on changes in health status or symptoms.

Educational Resources:

- Nutritional Education: Stay informed about heart-healthy eating through reputable sources and educational materials provided by healthcare providers.

- Cooking Classes: Consider participating in cooking classes focused on heart-healthy recipes and meal preparation.

Consideration of Medication Interactions:

- Discuss with Healthcare Providers: Some medications may interact with certain foods. Discuss potential interactions with healthcare providers and adjust the diet accordingly.

Collaboration with Healthcare Team:

- Open Communication: Communicate openly with healthcare providers about dietary habits, challenges, and any changes in symptoms.
- Regular Follow-ups: Regularly schedule follow-up appointments to

assess nutritional status and make necessary adjustments to the dietary plan.

Adhering to these dietary guidelines, combined with regular communication with healthcare providers, supports effective CHF management. A heart-healthy diet not only helps control symptoms but also contributes to overall cardiovascular well-being and an improved quality of life.

Exercise and Physical Activity

Physical activity is a crucial component of a comprehensive approach to managing Congestive Heart Failure (CHF). While individuals with CHF may face certain limitations, engaging in regular, tailored exercise can contribute to improved cardiovascular health, enhanced quality of life, and symptom management. Here are key considerations for incorporating exercise and physical activity into a CHF management plan:

Consultation with Healthcare Providers:

- Individualized Exercise Plan: Before starting any exercise regimen, consult with healthcare providers to create an individualized plan based on overall health, CHF severity, and potential limitations.

- Clearance for Exercise: Ensure medical clearance for exercise, as certain health conditions may require specific precautions or adjustments.

Types of Exercise:

- Aerobic Exercise: Moderate-intensity aerobic activities, such as walking, cycling, or swimming, can improve cardiovascular fitness and endurance.

- Strength Training: Incorporate light resistance training to improve muscle strength and support overall physical function.

- Flexibility and Balance Exercises: Include stretching and balance exercises to enhance flexibility and reduce the risk of falls.

Frequency and Duration:

- Gradual Progression: Begin with short sessions of exercise and gradually increase both frequency and duration as tolerated.
- Consistency: Aim for regular, consistent physical activity to maintain cardiovascular health.

Monitoring Intensity:

- Perceived Exertion: Use the Borg Rating of Perceived Exertion (RPE) scale to monitor exercise intensity. Individuals with CHF should aim for a moderate level of exertion.
- Heart Rate Monitoring: Some individuals may benefit from heart rate monitoring to ensure they stay within their target heart rate zone.

Tailoring Exercise to Symptoms:

- Listen to the Body: Pay attention to how the body responds to exercise. If experiencing increased fatigue, shortness of breath, or other symptoms, adjust the intensity or duration accordingly.
- Rest and Recovery: Allow for adequate rest and recovery between exercise sessions.

Incorporating Lifestyle Activities:

- Everyday Movement: Encourage daily physical activity through activities such as gardening, household chores, or taking the stairs.
- Functional Exercises: Focus on exercises that mimic daily activities to improve overall functional capacity.

Hydration:

- Maintain Fluid Balance: Stay hydrated by drinking water before, during, and after exercise. Be mindful of fluid restrictions if prescribed by healthcare providers.

Environmental Considerations:

- Temperature and Humidity: Exercise in a comfortable environment, considering factors like temperature and humidity, to prevent overheating or excessive strain on the cardiovascular system.

- Avoid Extreme Conditions: Minimize exposure to extreme weather conditions that may exacerbate symptoms.

Support Systems:

- Exercise Partners: Having a supportive exercise partner can enhance motivation and provide an added layer of safety.

- Supervised Programs: Consider participating in supervised exercise programs, such as cardiac rehabilitation, designed for individuals with heart conditions.

Regular Medical Check-ups:

- Monitoring Progress: Regularly update healthcare providers on exercise routines and progress during follow-up appointments.

- Adjustments as Needed: Based on health status, healthcare providers may adjust exercise recommendations to ensure safety and effectiveness.

Educational Resources:

- Educational Sessions: Attend educational sessions or classes on exercise and heart health to enhance understanding and motivation.
- Workshops on Safe Exercise Practices: Participate in workshops that focus on safe exercise practices for individuals with CHF.
- Adherence and Sustainability:
- Realistic Goals: Set realistic and achievable exercise goals that align with individual capabilities and health status.
- Long-Term Commitment: View exercise as a long-term commitment for cardiovascular health, symptom management, and overall well-being.

By integrating exercise into the management plan for CHF, individuals can experience numerous benefits, including improved cardiovascular fitness, enhanced energy levels, and better quality of life. Regular communication with healthcare providers ensures that exercise plans are tailored to individual needs and safety considerations.

Emotional Well-being

Emotional well-being is a vital aspect of managing Congestive Heart Failure (CHF), influencing overall health and quality of life. Living with a chronic condition like CHF can bring about various emotions, and addressing these feelings is essential for holistic care. Here are key considerations for promoting emotional well-being in individuals with CHF:

Open Communication:

- Discussing Feelings: Encourage open communication with healthcare providers, family members, and friends about emotional challenges related to CHF.

- Expressing Concerns: Share concerns, fears, or uncertainties to ensure a supportive environment.

Support Systems:

- Family and Friends: Cultivate a strong support network involving family, friends, and loved ones who understand and empathize with the challenges of living with CHF.

- Support Groups: Joining CHF support groups provides an opportunity to connect with others facing similar experiences, fostering understanding and shared coping strategies.

Education and Understanding:

- Knowledge Empowerment: Understanding the condition, its management, and treatment options empowers individuals, reducing anxiety and uncertainty.

- Access to Information: Utilize reputable sources and educational materials to stay informed about CHF and its impact on emotional well-being.

Mental Health Professionals:

- Counseling or Therapy: Seeking the assistance of mental health professionals, such as counselors or therapists, can provide valuable tools for coping with emotional challenges.
- Psychosocial Support: Mental health professionals can address stress, anxiety, and depression, contributing to improved overall well-being.

Mindfulness and Relaxation Techniques:

- Deep Breathing and Meditation: Practicing deep breathing exercises and meditation promotes relaxation, reducing stress and contributing to emotional balance.

- Mindfulness Practices: Engage in mindfulness techniques to stay present and focused, preventing excessive worry about the future.

Maintaining a Positive Outlook:

- Focusing on Achievements: Celebrate personal achievements, no matter how small, and maintain a positive outlook on progress and resilience.

- Setting Realistic Goals: Establish realistic goals that align with individual capabilities, fostering a sense of accomplishment.

Adapting to Lifestyle Changes:

- Adjustment Period: Recognize that adapting to lifestyle changes may take time. Be patient and acknowledge the efforts made in managing CHF.
- Flexibility: Embrace flexibility in daily routines and activities, allowing for adjustments as needed.

Addressing Sleep Disturbances:

- Quality Sleep: Prioritize good sleep hygiene to promote restful sleep. Addressing sleep disturbances positively impacts emotional well-being.
- Consulting Healthcare Providers: If sleep problems persist, consult healthcare providers for guidance and potential interventions.

Engaging in Hobbies and Interests:

- Leisure Activities: Participate in hobbies and activities that bring joy and relaxation. Engaging in enjoyable pursuits contributes to emotional well-being.

- Social Engagement: Stay socially connected with loved ones and friends through shared activities and interests.

Goal Setting and Planning:

- Short-Term and Long-Term Goals: Establish both short-term and long-term goals, creating a sense of purpose and direction.

- Involving Healthcare Providers: Involve healthcare providers in goal-setting discussions to ensure alignment with overall health objectives.

Regular Medical Check-ups:

- Monitoring Emotional Well-being: Regularly discuss emotional well-being during medical check-ups. Healthcare providers can offer additional support or referrals if needed.

Empowerment and Self-Care:

- Active Participation: Actively participate in the management of CHF, taking ownership of self-care and treatment adherence.

- Self-Compassion: Practice self-compassion and acknowledge the strength and resilience demonstrated in the face of CHF.

Promoting emotional well-being in CHF management involves a holistic approach, encompassing psychological, social, and behavioral aspects. Creating a supportive environment, seeking professional assistance when needed, and fostering a positive mindset contribute to a comprehensive strategy for emotional well-being in individuals living with CHF.

Conclusion

In conclusion, living with Congestive Heart Failure (CHF) requires a multifaceted approach that encompasses medical management, lifestyle adjustments, and attention to emotional well-being. This book has explored various facets of CHF, providing insights into understanding the condition, its causes, and the importance of managing it effectively.

From the significance of lifestyle changes and dietary guidelines to the role of exercise, surgical interventions, and emotional well-being, individuals with CHF can navigate their daily lives with a proactive and informed mindset. Medications, diagnostic tests, and treatment options have been discussed, emphasizing the collaborative effort between healthcare providers and patients in achieving optimal outcomes.

As we acknowledge the challenges that CHF presents, it's equally important to highlight the resilience and strength demonstrated by individuals facing this condition. Empowerment through education, support from healthcare teams, and the embrace of lifestyle modifications contribute to a better quality of life for those living with CHF.

The journey with CHF involves ongoing adaptation, regular medical follow-ups, and a commitment to self-care. By fostering open communication, building strong support networks, and staying informed about the latest developments in CHF management, individuals can lead fulfilling lives while effectively managing their health.

This book serves as a resource for individuals with CHF, their caregivers, and healthcare professionals, offering valuable insights into the comprehensive approach needed to address the complexities of this condition. As we look toward the future, advancements in research and healthcare practices will continue to shape the landscape of CHF management, offering hope and improved outcomes for individuals living with this cardiovascular condition.

Living Well with CHF

Living Well with CHF" is not just a goal but an achievable reality with a proactive and informed approach. Here are key principles to guide individuals in thriving while managing Congestive Heart Failure (CHF):

Education and Awareness:

- Empowerment through Knowledge: Understanding CHF, its causes, and management options empowers individuals to actively participate in their care.
- Continuous Learning: Stay informed about the latest developments in CHF management through reputable sources and ongoing communication with healthcare providers.

Medical Adherence:

- Consistent Medication Use: Adhering to prescribed medications as directed by healthcare providers is essential for symptom control and overall health.
- Open Communication: Communicate openly about any challenges or concerns related to medications, ensuring adjustments when necessary.

Lifestyle Modifications:

- Heart-Healthy Eating: Embrace a low-sodium, heart-healthy diet rich in fruits, vegetables, and whole grains.
- Regular Exercise: Engage in tailored exercise programs to improve cardiovascular fitness and overall well-being.
- Fluid and Sodium Management: Monitor fluid intake and adhere to

sodium restrictions as advised by healthcare providers.

Emotional Well-being:

- Open Dialogue: Foster open communication with healthcare providers, family, and support networks about emotional challenges.

- Mental Health Support: Seek support from mental health professionals when needed to address stress, anxiety, or depression.

Regular Medical Check-ups:

- Proactive Monitoring: Attend regular follow-up appointments for ongoing assessment of CHF management and adjustments to the care plan.

- Collaboration with Healthcare Team: Actively participate in discussions with healthcare providers to ensure a coordinated and personalized approach to care.

Support Networks:

- Family and Friends: Cultivate strong relationships with supportive family and friends who understand the challenges of living with CHF.

- Support Groups: Participate in CHF support groups to connect with others facing similar experiences, fostering a sense of community.

Adaptability:

- Flexibility in Lifestyle: Embrace adaptability in daily routines, adjusting to changes in health status or treatment plans.

- Resilience: Cultivate resilience in the face of challenges, recognizing the progress made and focusing on achievable goals.

Holistic Self-Care:

- Mind-Body Connection: Recognize the interplay between physical and emotional well-being, emphasizing holistic self-care.

- Prioritize Self-Care Practices: Engage in activities that promote relaxation, enjoyment, and overall well-being.

Goal Setting:

- Realistic Goals: Set realistic short-term and long-term goals, celebrating achievements and milestones along the way.

- Collaboration with Healthcare Providers: Involve healthcare providers in goal-setting discussions to ensure alignment with overall health objectives.

Living in the Present:

- Mindfulness: Practice mindfulness to stay present, appreciating the moments and experiences that contribute to a fulfilling life.
- Gratitude: Cultivate a sense of gratitude for the support received, achievements made, and the opportunity to lead a meaningful life.

Living well with CHF is not just about managing symptoms; it's about embracing life with purpose, resilience, and a commitment to holistic well-being. By integrating these principles into daily life, individuals with CHF can thrive, finding joy and fulfillment on their journey.

Encouragement and Hope

In the face of Congestive Heart Failure (CHF), finding encouragement and holding onto hope is paramount. Here are uplifting words to inspire you

Resilience:

- Embrace the strength within you. Every step you take in managing CHF is a testament to your resilience and courage.

Progress, Not Perfection:

- Celebrate the small victories, recognizing that progress, no matter how gradual, is a significant achievement on this journey.

Community Support:

- You are not alone. Surround yourself with a supportive community of healthcare professionals, friends, and family who stand by you on this path.

Adaptability:

- Life with CHF may bring changes, but your ability to adapt and find new ways to enjoy each day showcases your resilience and creativity.

Hope Springs Eternal:

- In every sunrise and new day, find hope. The future holds possibilities for advancements in treatments and continued improvements in CHF management.

Courage in Challenges:

- Every challenge you face is an opportunity to showcase your courage.

You have the strength to overcome obstacles and emerge stronger.

Shared Experiences:

- Connect with others who understand your journey. Shared experiences create a sense of solidarity and provide comfort in knowing you are not alone.

Tomorrow's Opportunities:

- Tomorrow brings new opportunities for progress and joy. Approach each day with optimism, and look forward to the possibilities ahead.

Inner Strength:

- Your inner strength is a guiding force. Tap into it, and let it empower you to face each day with determination and grace.

Purpose and Meaning:

- Find purpose and meaning in your journey. Your experiences with CHF contribute to a narrative of strength, resilience, and the pursuit of well-being.

Healthcare Partnership:

- Your partnership with healthcare providers is a beacon of hope. Together, you work towards managing CHF and achieving the best possible outcomes.

Joy in Moments:

- Cherish the moments of joy and connection. Whether big or small, these moments contribute to a life rich in experiences and meaning.

Remember, your journey with CHF is unique, and you are the hero of your story. Each day presents an opportunity for growth, resilience, and a renewed sense of hope. In the midst of challenges, find encouragement in the progress you make and the support that surrounds you. You are stronger than you know, and hope is a guiding light on your path.

<u>Bonus</u>

Ten Easy Steps To Living A Fulfilled life With CHF

Living a fulfilled life with Congestive Heart Failure (CHF) involves a holistic approach that encompasses physical, emotional, and social well-being. Here are ten easy steps to enhance your quality of life while managing CHF:

Educate Yourself:

- Stay Informed: Learn about CHF, its symptoms, and management strategies. Knowledge empowers you to actively participate in your care and make informed decisions.

Healthy Eating Habits:

- Balanced Diet: Adopt a heart-healthy diet with an emphasis on fruits, vegetables, whole grains, and lean proteins. Limit sodium intake and practice portion control.

Regular Exercise:

- Tailored Physical Activity: Engage in regular, moderate exercise tailored to your abilities. Consult with healthcare providers to create a safe and effective exercise plan.

Medication Adherence:

- Consistent Medication Use: Take prescribed medications as directed by healthcare providers. Adhering to your medication regimen is crucial for symptom control.

Emotional Well-being:

- Open Communication: Discuss your emotions and concerns with healthcare providers, friends, and family. Seek support when needed, and consider counseling to address stress and anxiety.

Build a Support Network:

- Family and Friends: Cultivate strong relationships with supportive friends and family members. Their understanding and encouragement can make a significant difference.

Regular Check-ups:

- Routine Medical Visits: Attend regular follow-up appointments with healthcare providers. Regular check-ups help monitor your health status and ensure timely adjustments to your care plan.

Set Realistic Goals:

- Achievable Milestones: Establish realistic short-term and long-term goals. Celebrate achievements, no matter how small, and use them as motivation for further progress.

Engage in Hobbies:

- Pursue Enjoyable Activities: Participate in hobbies and activities that bring joy and fulfillment. Engaging in things you love contributes to a positive mindset.

Practice Gratitude:

- Focus on the Positive: Cultivate a mindset of gratitude. Acknowledge the positive aspects of your life and express appreciation for the support you receive.

Remember, each step is a part of the larger journey toward a fulfilled life with CHF. By taking these simple yet impactful steps, you can actively shape your daily experiences, enhance your overall well-being, and find joy in the journey of living well with CHF.

7 Days Meal Plan

Creating a balanced and heart-healthy meal plan for Congestive Heart Failure (CHF) involves incorporating nutrient-dense foods, controlling sodium intake, and maintaining proper portion sizes. Here's a sample 7-day meal plan to get you started:

Day 1:

Breakfast:

- Oatmeal with sliced strawberries and a sprinkle of chia seeds.
- A cup of green tea.

Lunch:

- Grilled chicken breast with quinoa.
- Steamed broccoli and a side of mixed greens.

- Fresh fruit salad.

Dinner:

- Baked salmon with a lemon-dill sauce.
- Brown rice pilaf.
- Roasted asparagus.

Day 2:

Breakfast:

- Greek yogurt parfait with blueberries and a handful of almonds.
- Herbal tea.

Lunch:

- Lentil soup with whole-grain crackers.
- Spinach and cherry tomato salad with a light vinaigrette.
- Sliced melon.

Dinner:

- Grilled tilapia with a citrus salsa.
- Quinoa and black bean salad.

- Steamed green beans.

Day 3:

Breakfast:

- Whole-grain toast with avocado.

- Fresh orange slices.

- Low-sodium vegetable juice.

Lunch:

- Turkey and vegetable wrap with whole-grain tortilla.

- Mixed greens salad with a balsamic vinaigrette.

- Apple slices.

Dinner:

- Stir-fried tofu with broccoli and bell peppers.

- Brown rice.

- Sliced mango for dessert.

Day 4:

Breakfast:

- Smoothie with banana, spinach, Greek yogurt, and a dash of cinnamon.
- Whole-grain toast with almond butter.

Lunch:

- Quinoa and black bean bowl with diced tomatoes and avocado.
- Side of sliced cucumber.
- Fresh berries.

Dinner:

- Grilled chicken Caesar salad with a light dressing.
- Roasted sweet potatoes.
- Steamed asparagus.

Day 5:

Breakfast:

- Scrambled eggs with spinach and tomatoes.

- Whole-grain English muffin.
- Freshly squeezed orange juice.

Lunch:

- Chickpea salad with cherry tomatoes, cucumber, and feta.
- Whole-grain pita bread.
- Sliced pineapple.

Dinner:

- Baked cod with a lemon-herb crust.
- Quinoa pilaf with mixed vegetables.
- Steamed broccoli.

Day 6:

Breakfast:

- Cottage cheese with sliced peaches.
- Whole-grain toast with jam.
- Green tea.

Lunch:

- Whole-grain pasta with marinara sauce and grilled vegetables.
- Spinach and walnut salad.
- Mixed fruit bowl.

Dinner:

- Turkey meatballs with tomato sauce.
- Whole-grain couscous.
- Roasted Brussels sprouts.

Day 7:

Breakfast:

- Overnight oats with mixed berries and a drizzle of honey.
- Herbal tea.

Lunch:

- Quinoa and chickpea-stuffed bell peppers.

- Mixed greens with a light olive oil dressing.
- Sliced kiwi.

Dinner:

- Grilled shrimp skewers with a garlic-lime marinade.
- Brown rice.
- Steamed green beans.

Remember to adjust portion sizes based on individual dietary needs and consult with healthcare providers or a nutritionist for personalized guidance. Additionally, drink plenty of water throughout the day to stay hydrated.